Light Ten Up!

Ten Lifestyle Essentials to *Glow By*

by

Danielle Day

For Megan, Greg, and Anessa.
Thank you for always helping me find my way.

And a special shout-out to
Don Miguel Ruiz, Jr. for codifying
Ritual, Order and Ceremony in The Four Agreements,

and to Kinetix for "Genuine Human Connection"
and the job that saved my life from 2008-2010.

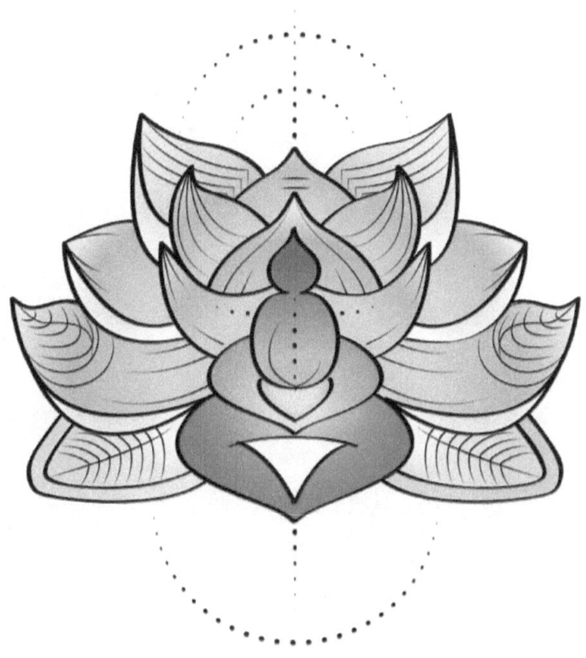

Table of Contents

GIVE IT UP!
Acknowledgments

I owe a huge debt of gratitude to Dr Mark Dedomenico of PRO Sports Club, Redmond, Washington, Founder of the 20/20 Lifestyles Program. Thank you from the bottom of my heart for your good work, and for the chance to learn so much in your clinical weight loss program. As a personal trainer and 20/20 Lifestyles Certified Coach, I learned everything I know about anatomy, physiology, metabolic diseases, and PRO BEST. I still recall everything from your lectures. It is my goal to showcase the knowledge, skills and abilities I developed all throughout my time with you from 2003 to 2008. Going on to Kinetix, serving Starbucks Corporate Fitness clientele alongside the superstars I'd met at PRO, was so fulfilling too. I met my best friend at PRO, and I networked with the greatest cast members of all time. I became a group fitness instructor, a USAT Level 1 triathlon coach, a yoga teacher, and ultimately an Ironman Triathlete and yoga teacher trainer, all because of PRO SPORTS CLUB.

*Fun Fact: I have a flashbulb memory of being a child in the 1970's, watching television, in Bellevue, Washington, and **seeing you** in a commercial, holding the plate of Mission Pasta, saying, **"From our family to yours**…" YES, I totally remember lying on my tummy, looking into the eyes of a blonde, young future Doctor Mark. It's amazing that one day you, the spokesperson for the Mission Pasta family, would become the heart surgeon who wrote the original paper on children's open-heart surgery….and my boss. I was five years old when I saw you on TV.*

*In 2003, I was the very last personal trainer hired at PRO, without a four-year degree in exercise physiology. **I am so grateful the Universe sent me to work at PRO. Thank You!***

BUCKLE UP!
Let's Get Started

Hello and welcome! Thank you for the chance to tell you about a system of living that I have developed over a twenty-year career in fitness. *Light Ten Up! Ten Lifestyle Essentials to Glow By* is the sum total of everything I have learned, helping people get into the best shape of their lives. As a lifestyle coach, my journey is to support *your* journey. *Light Ten Up! Ten Lifestyle Essentials to Glow By* is the book I wrote because I absolutely had to. I wrote this book because I could not bear it *not* being in the world another minute longer. Thank you for taking a look. This book is my testament to the healing power of nutrition, fitness and genuine human connection. It's my honor to share what I've learned.

A little background before we get started on this path together. I was a career social worker for ten years, but ultimately chose instead to work at the gym. I took my social work skills and pursued fitness because I believe self-care is at the heart of happiness. In 2002, I became a certified personal trainer and group fitness instructor, going on to accomplish my personal goals, and those of my beloved clients. My focus became training clinical weight loss patients to compete in marathons and Ironman triathlons. My passion for genuine human connection and love of yoga led me to my career as a certified yoga instructor and yoga teacher trainer.

It is my intention to share the lifestyle essentials that I have practiced in times of great purpose and clarity. At times in my life, I have been at my absolute best balancing nutrition, fitness and lifestyle choices, such as dining out and alcohol. At other times, I was not prioritizing this self-care. To this I like to say, *I got the results I earned.*

Please know, Friend. The object of *Light Ten Up!* is to offer you the strategies that are finally helping me live in optimal wellness, optimal fun, and optimal healthy happiness! Before we get started, I want to share a little more about what makes this system unique. I spent ten years as a social worker, ten years as a fitness trainer, and ten years teaching yoga teachers how to guide beautiful, life-affirming yoga classes. This thirty-year sum total of knowledge, skills and abilities boils down to my secrets for success: *Ritual, Order and Ceremony*.

Friends, throughout this system, you will notice these three shining stars that guide us.

- Ritual - Performing the <u>same</u> tasks every day.
- Order - Following a system <u>by the book</u>.
- Ceremony - <u>Imbuing the ordinary with extraordinary gratitude</u>, mindful of the blessings that are upon us.

To me, there is no such thing as an ordinary moment, an ordinary day, or an ordinary thought. People are magical, magnetic creatures who create their own lives, circumstances and surroundings. Belief in the potential of every living being, reverence for the beauty of existence, and an absolute passion for being alive are *choices*. Eating, drinking, moving and thinking are all *choices*. The sum total of our physical, mental and emotional well-being are all connected.

So are we. Let's start the journey together.

FIRE IT UP!
Introduction

Under the surface of your skin beats the heart of a champion, who is ready to shine. You really are Enough. That is true. If you also want to fit into your favorite clothes and reboot your lifestyle, then this is the book for you.

I created *Light Ten Up! Ten Lifestyle Essentials to Glow By* to codify the ten lifestyle essentials that keep me on the path toward my best. I'm excited to share them with you. Please know, I am not a nutritionist, but I have thirty years of experience coaching my clients to their best and most accountable selves. I am here to help you choose your ideal routine, keeping some of the foods you love, while balancing calorie density and macronutrients to unlock your full potential.

My love of yoga and strength training inspired the fitness routines I have created. These routines are safe, effective and they are fun! Incorporating my years of education and experience, I have developed these routines, teaching students since 2003. My specialty is folding my science-based knowledge of musculature and anatomy into my exercise programming.

I look forward to helping you online in my YouTube classes. In this special library of archived live classes, you will find everything you need. Supporting your journey is my passion. I look forward to helping you out in this book, over the internet, as well as through my podcast, *Light Not Might* (a great screen-free indulgence!).

LIGHT TEN UP!
The System

1.   Wake Up!

   1st Thing's First: Plan your nutrition & exercise for the day.

2.   Pump it Up!

   2 Days to Lift Weights: Tuesday & Thursday strength training.

3.   Open Up!

   3 Days to Yoga: Monday, Wednesday & Friday Yoga.

4.   Drink Up!

   4 Liters of Water: Proper hydration supports weight loss.

5.   Tighten Up!

   5 Min. Lymphatic Massage: Dry brushing for detoxification.

6.   Thumbs Up!

   6th Day Selfie: Saturday is for selfies, stats & for celebration.

7.   Stock Up!

   7 Days of Dinners: Suppertime, planned & purchased weekly.

8.   Rest Up!

   8 Hours of Sleep: Sleep balances hormones for weight loss.

9.   Light it Up!

   9 Minutes of Tai Chi'll: My meditation & movement practice.

10.   Step it Up!

   10,000 Steps Per Day: Minimum for weight loss & maintenance.

WAKE UP!
TEN-et One

1st Thing's First

The first lifestyle essential of *Light Ten Up!* is the first step of every day. I call it *First Thing's First* because this is your mantra for self-care. You must put your needs first as you schedule your day around work, family, and other commitments. Like the oxygen mask speech on the airplane, you must attend to your life saving efforts first, so that you can assist others well.

This is a 20-minute window every morning devoted to planning. Each new day is the blessing of 24 hours you get to use in order to move closer to your goal. This first essential step sets the stage for the entire day. By performing the rituals of this step, you can be certain that you will move forward towards your goal. This first step is a chance to choose with clarity and purpose what you will accomplish.

This lifestyle essential is a daily ritual, taking approximately twenty minutes to plan everything you will eat, drink and do before the day begins. Again, think ritual, order and ceremony. Take twenty minutes in a quiet space, with your coffee or tea, and set the stage, set the tone, set your inTENtions for the best day ever.

I recommend that you use an app such as Nutritionix to record your dinner plan first, then add your coffee or tea, breakfast, lunch, and snack notions. Tally the choices. Notice the calorie density, nutrient density, and adjust your choices accordingly. Nutritionix is great to use because you can get an immediate summary of your macros, nutrients and calories. I love tweaking my choices first thing in the morning for the perfect daily plan. The app is like having your own dietician explaining in real time how you can get more protein, fewer carbs, and enough iron, calcium and vitamins A and C for your day. Make this habit your first step every day. Then, enjoy planning your dinners. Make it fun, and the routine becomes second nature.

<u>Checklist for TEN-et One: WAKE UP!</u>

- Weigh yourself first thing in the morning and write it down in your journal. Every day.
- Start your coffee or tea and pour the four liters of water that you'll drink that day into a fancy spa jug. Add a shake of pink Himalayan sea salt for electrolytes. Please!
- Look at your day. Plan your workouts to fit in with your schedule, meetings and appointments. You are carving out the time to exercise as a high priority.
- Open your nutrition tracker app and budget your calories and macro goals.
- Enter into the nutrition tracker what you plan to eat for dinner that night first.
- Identify your snacks of choice.
- Enter in your breakfast and lunch choices next. Your goal is to choose what you want to eat most of all, and then to make it work within the other choices *before the day begins*.
- Throughout the day, refer to your plan as a guide. Choose the foods that fit into your plan, and adjust as needed throughout the day,

Choose a healthy range of macronutrients.

Carbohydrates should be 20-40%, Protein 30-40%, and fats 20-50% for best results. Aim for a range. Be flexible. Choose no fewer than 1,200 calories for women and no fewer than 1,800 calories for men. I use the tracker Nutritionix.

Keep it simple. I like to refer to the theme song from the 90's television show Frasier: **Tossed salads and scrambled eggs!** I eat eggs for breakfast, and salads (or dinner leftovers) for lunch every day. I weigh and measure everything and always plan around my favorites first. The secret here is to plan ahead for the entire day, every morning. Keep track of your calories, and you will be on track to your best!

I personally target 1,200 calories a day, with 50 percent of the calories coming from fat. I eat 25% protein, and I split the other 25% between carbohydrates and alcohol. My goal is to keep my carbs at 20-50 grams, depending on my cardio for the day. Example: I am training for a marathon. Sunday is for my weekly long run. Therefore, I budget for fifty grams of carbohydrate on the day before (DATE NIGHT). On days when I am less active, I keep the carbs to twenty grams and enjoy one to two servings of alcohol. **Twenty is plenty**. That is my mantra.

PUMP IT UP!
TEN-et Two

2 Days to Lift Weights

The second lifestyle essential of *Light Ten Up!* is strength training for 60 minutes, twice a week.

I have created a 60-minute workout for Tuesdays and Thursdays for all major muscle groups. This workout includes 2 sets of 12-15 repetitions, using simple dumbbells and a yoga mat. Make this plan work for you at home! Find a space that feels comfortable and motivating. Lifting weights at home twice a week can help boost your metabolism, improve your vital capacity and tone your muscles. My YouTube videos (OpenUpWithDanielleDay) will walk you through these simple, safe exercises. The American College of Sports Medicine recommends that you lift weights twice a week for 8-10 major muscle groups. Choose weights that get you to volitional fatigue: that moment where you want to do the last rep but cannot do so with proper form.

Strength training provides an immediate boost to your resting metabolic rate. This routine leads to EPOC, or Excess Post-Exercise Oxygen Consumption, from your very first workout! This means that your body will burn more calories, as you recover from your bout of strength training. Good job!

Ready? Let's begin.

<u>Checklist for TEN-et Two: PUMP IT UP!</u>

This workout includes 2 sets of 12-15 repetitions using hand weights. Select dumb bells that are Heavy: 12-20 pounds, Medium: 8 to 12 pounds, and Light: 2 to 5 pounds.

<u>SET 1</u>

Squats, with one heavy dumb bell.

Pushups (from your knees works just fine).

<u>SET 2</u>

Lunges with **Bicep Curls**, alternating legs, using two medium dumb bells.

Deadlifts with one heavy dumb bell.

<u>SET 3</u>

Chest Presses, (utilizing cushions or a weight bench) with two heavy dumb bells,

One-Arm Rows, alternating arms, with one heavy dumb bell.

<u>SET 4</u>

Single-leg Rear-Delt Flys with two medium-sized dumb bells.

Overhead Presses with High Kicks, using the same medium-sized dumb bells.

<u>SET 5</u>

Tricep Extensions in Tree pose from Yoga, right leg, using 2 light dumb bells.

Lateral Raises in Tree pose, left leg, using the same 2 light dumb bells.

<u>CORE</u>

I recommend the great ab workout video on YouTube called "**8-Minute Abs**" from 1993.

NOTES:

Remember to exhale on exertion, and to keep your spine in neutral position, lifting with your legs, and keeping your eyes on the horizon.

Of course, make sure you are healthy for exercise and work into the routine gradually. Again, please find my videos on my YouTube channel - OpenUpWithDanielleDay. These videos are a great way for me to guide you on your time!

OPEN UP!
TEN-et Three

3 Days to Yoga

The third lifestyle essential of *Light Ten Up!* is Yoga, performed three times a week for 60 minutes. My YouTube video, **"Hatha Yoga Class - Leaving Bikram"** is the best class for you to use, along with the entire *Light Ten Up!* system. I call this lifestyle essential "Open Up!", because that is the name of my company: Open Up Yoga, LLC.

Three times a week, on Monday, Wednesday and Friday, the ritual of this 60-minute yoga practice called Hatha Fusion will change your life. By repeating this same class each time, three times a week, you will improve agility, balance and coordination. You will observe, over time, your abilities blossom as your body adapts and changes. This class features all-levels instruction and is perfect for every shape and ability.

Whether you are a "yoga person" or not, I am sharing with you this lifestyle essential. Yoga is the most effective healthy habit of all. Yoga is nature's most comprehensive system for wellness. Yes, you will burn calories. But more to the point, you will rinse your organs, improve range of motion, recover quickly from any stress and sleep way better.

*I am obsessed with my yoga class **"Leaving Bikram."** I personally do this class for 60 minutes every day. I am on a 365-day challenge that I began October 10, 2020 and in the first two months I lost 17 pounds. In this particular video, I walk you through all the moves. It's 60 minutes of all-levels guidance. I encourage you to practice three times a week for best results. Stick with it! It will work wonders for your mind, body and soul.*

If you choose another activity for cardio (like Peloton, elliptical, biking, hiking, running, dancing, etc.) enjoy it for an hour, and do it thrice weekly for an hour. Please consider that yoga and getting 10,000 steps a day is Enough. I enjoy running and cycling and hiking too, but when I selected the recommendations for Light Ten Up! I selected yoga as the superior choice. When I complete my next marathon, I choose to maintain my results just like I am recommending here in this book. For the rest of my life, I know I can maintain a healthy weight and a happy life with these ten essentials.

As I glow older, running is not sustainable for my knees. Yoga and walking 10,000 steps and, of course, Tai Chi'll will never hurt me. Or You! □

Let's Glow Old Together!

<u>Checklist for TEN-et Three: OPEN UP!</u>

- Subscribe to my YouTube channel ***Open Up! with Danielle Day***. There, you will find many resources if you are new or are returning to Yoga.
- Use a yoga mat and consider using a mirror so you can see yourself.
- Use the same outfit every day, or set out your workout clothes the night before, so you won't have another thing to remember.
- Pro Tip: Keep coconut oil in a mini crockpot. Plug it in ten minutes before your practice. This ritual offers a way to spread warm, nutty goodness on your skin so you can slip easily in and out of poses. The warmth feels like a hug. Enjoy!
- Put your gear in a quiet space where you might also hang a plant, flowers or a picture of your goal. Your yoga space should make you feel quiet and peaceful. Pets welcome!

Of course, make sure you are healthy for exercise and work into the routine gradually. I'm looking forward to supporting your efforts on the mat. Yoga is the best practice for rinsing your organs, supporting your spine, and encouraging agility, balance and coordination. Enjoy the process. Be gentle on yourself. I'll see you on YouTube and we can practice together!

DRINK UP!
TEN-et Four

4 Liters of Water

The fourth lifestyle essential of *Light Ten Up!* is critical. Drink 4 liters of water daily. Proper hydration works wonders for every system in your body. Drinking the proper amount of water promotes weight loss, helping to address bloating caused by stress, and from eating processed, refined foods. Blood pressure and insulin sensitivity are also enhanced with proper hydration, as well as recovery from exercise. Fatigue is often a sign of poor hydration.

If the target of 4 liters feels random, let's calculate how much you personally will need. Take the number of pounds you weighed this morning and convert the number from pounds to ounces. Then divide that number by half. *This is the amount of water you need to keep your kidneys healthy.* Add 12 more ounces for every dehydrating beverage you drink, such as coffee or alcohol.

Example: I weighed 164 today, so 164 ounces divided by two is 82. I did yoga, so that's another 12 ounces for 94 ounces total, and I walked 45 minutes, so adding another 12 ounces, that's now 106 ounces. I had two cups of coffee, so adding 24 more, we are now at 130 ounces. 135 ounces is 4 Liters, so this is just about perfect.

<u>Checklist for TEN-et Four: DRINK UP!</u>

- If you are working from home today, or if you have a desk space to put a party jug, I really recommend the kind of jug that you see at the spa. 4 Liters is pretty standard.

- Fill the jug first thing in the morning, while coffee is brewing. I like to add a bottle of Hint Water. I only use one Hint water per day, to keep my plastic waste to a minimum, but oh my it tastes great to add the cherry flavored water to my plain, filtered tap water.

- Add one crystal of unrefined Pink Himalayan sea salt to your water, PLEASE A single crystal is all it takes to provide sodium, potassium, iron, and magnesium. Unrefined pink Himalayan sea salt is the purest form of electrolytes, in the most bioavailable form. Your body needs sodium and potassium to function. Gatorade and other electrolyte supplements are costly, with additives such as sugar. You will not taste the salt in your water when you use a single crystal. (You will avert hyponatremia, the toxic desalinization of your bloodstream.)

- Supplementing with electrolytes is not the same thing as eating salty foods. Don't worry. You will not retain water by supplementing with pink Himalayan sea salt.

- Employ the ritual, order and ceremony to filling your spa jug in the morning. Think about how healthy and energetic every cell in your body will feel with this hydration.

- I like to say the mantra *"Pour the Four"* as I fill the jug, adding a bottle of Hint brand water and a shake of pink Himalayan sea salt. I recommend Himala brand of pink Himalayan sea salt, but any unrefined pink Himalayan sea salt will suffice. Friends, hyponatremia (loss of sodium) and hypokalemia (loss of potassium) are deadly. Please never consume large amounts of pure water without these electrolytes. Also, please consult your doctor for advice regarding your own needs. Blood pressure concerns, pre-diabetes and other metabolic syndromes need special attention. Thank you.

TIGHTEN UP!
TEN-et Five

5 Min. Lymphatic Massage

The fifth lifestyle essential of *Light Ten Up!* is also magical, in that you see results almost immediately. A five-minute practice of lymphatic massage in the shower is for self-myofascial release. "Myo" means muscle, and fascia is a network of connective tissue so pervasive throughout your body, that if we took everything off of you except the fascia, we would still know it was you. The relationship between muscle and fascia determines everything from the range of motion around your joints, to detoxification in your tissues. Adipose tissue, or stored fat, and your individual collagen structure determines the appearance of any cellulite or dimply skin. Reducing puffiness through dry brushing of the skin, or lymphatic massage, as you'll learn here, is possible.

Your lymphatic system is a key feature of your immune system. Moving lymph around your body depends upon the milking action of skeletal muscle fibers by way of hatha yoga poses, or lymphatic massage. There is no other pump for lymph to move around your body. A spa tech can administer lymphatic massage, or you can take matters into your own hands. Let's find out how.

This lifestyle essential is a five- minute daily practice you can do in the shower. This works miracles with weight loss, improving the appearance of your arms, legs and midriff. You'll have the most success if you can set a timer when you are in the shower and stick to the five-minute duration.

I like having my Alexa speaker set five minutes for me, so I don't have to guess the time.

Again, lymphatic massage by dry brushing the skin promotes the circulation of interstitial fluids that accumulate within the adipose tissues and fascia under the skin. Fascia is the magical lining of every nook and cranny in your body. Within the fascial planes, we can accumulate toxins and retain fluids. The dimply effect on our thighs and legs and midriff can drastically change with regular lymphatic massage, such as dry brushing. This is very motivating, as you begin to see and feel the difference!

Check out my class on *YouTube*, regarding how to do this step.

<u>Checklist for TEN-et Five: TIGHTEN UP!</u>

- Get a dry brush. Look for them in the wellness section at Whole Foods. Also get exfoliating bath gloves and a pedicure tool for the bottoms of your feet, along with Dr Bronner's soap. It's the purest.

You can enjoy warm water for this step. If you like, you can alternate hot and cooler water to promote circulation, like a Scandinavian sauna! You can also do the dry brushing before you even step into the shower, for even better results. Start at your feet, brushing all the way up your legs to your groin. Then go from hands to arm pits, and tummy to sternum.

- In the shower, starting at your feet, take the gloves and massage the tops and bottoms of your ankles then, as though you were pulling up panty hose, run your gloves up to your groin. This inner thigh line is where the lymph nodes are. You are pulling interstitial fluid to these ducts.
- Work from your arms, from your wrists to your armpits, working to empty at the neckline nodes. Work last from your navel to your collarbone, from tummy to sternum.
- Run the dry brush in the same way you used the gloves, finishing with the backs of your thighs, running upwards, several times from knee crease to gluteal fold. This works like magic. Yoga, hydration, strength training and nutrition, combined with dry brushing will unlock amazing results. *Can you imagine the difference you will see and feel? You deserve these kinds of results. I'm excited for you!*

PS. A note of gratitude. Lymphatic Drainage Technology was invented in Germany to reduce dimples under the skin. This process is a secret, taught to me by my own lymphatic drainage technician. I used to attend LDT sessions at a spa, during which an electrode wand is passed over the tissues. According to my technician, Hatha Yoga, combined with the dry brushing techniques I am teaching you, combine to replicate this effect. How wonderful, to reap the benefits at home, for free! Any dimply appearance under your skin can be ironed out with these practices. Everyone has a different level of collagen density under their skin, but everyone can see the results from self-myofascial release practices like dry brushing.

THUMBS UP!
TEN-et Six

6th Day Selfie

The sixth lifestyle essential of *Light Ten Up!* is a weekly check-in with your progress. Take a progress photo every Saturday morning. At first, this might not feel very fun, but trust me, it is important. After a few weeks of this practice, you will see the results clearly!

Along the lines of ritual, order and ceremony, taking a progress picture every Saturday morning will enable you to celebrate your results. Celebration is a vital component of living. The ceremony and fanfare around acknowledging your accomplishments tells your brain that you are on the right track. More good results come soon after.

Think of it like this. When you eat junk food, your body prepares to receive nutrients. When empty calories come in, cellular sensitivity to insulin wears down over time. Diabetes can occur, when such insulin resistance goes unabated. That's kind of what happens in life too.

When you work so hard without ever stopping and patting yourself on the back, nourishing your soul, pausing to reflect and to feel grateful, your body never gets to assimilate the new reality. Your brain never gets to assimilate the new reality. You wait to feel the accomplishment *on a day that never comes*. Ritual, order and ceremony, like a Saturday selfie, will help you to celebrate every step of the way.

Of course, you will also hold yourself accountable to your goals. But please do not miss the point. In an effort to get to your best, take shame out of the game. *No amount of waking up angry at yourself again is ever going to lead to lasting change. If you tell yourself you're messing up all the time, why in the world would you stick with anything? Self-Talk is my coaching area of expertise. Thank you for listening.*

The Saturday selfie is also a great time to record your current weight, and to check in with your coach, or someone who will help keep you on plan. If you are working with me, this is the weekly time where we will talk about what you feel is working and address any challenges you are experiencing. *Prepare to open with what you are doing right. Not what you are doing wrong. Gratitude brings more results than shame.*

If you are doing this program independently, think of the Saturday Selfie as something to post or share with your best friend. It's so fun, doing a challenge together. I am on a group chat with friends. We use a spreadsheet to log our alcohol intake, workouts and progress. I have fun friends who rally to help keep each other on track. It feels good to post progress.

Throughout my personal training career, I have taught my clients the mantra, "*Listen to Your Pants*". When what you see on the scale does not match the progress you are feeling in your body, trying on clothing can be very illuminating. Similarly, taking a photo in the same outfit every Saturday can show you what you really have accomplished!

<u>Checklist for TEN-et Six: THUMBS UP!</u>

- Take a weekly progress photo in the same outfit each weekend and record your weight.
- Check in with your coach or your accountability partner.
- Set reasonable goals. A healthy target for weight loss is to lose a half a pound to a pound per week.

Losing one pound of fat means you burned an excess of 3,500 calories over intake.

Saturday is probably DATE NIGHT, so it's great to get your stats "out there" and to enjoy yourself.

DATE NIGHT implies that you are enjoying some in-TEN-tional relaxation. Whether you are on an actual date, or just relaxing with pets, family or by yourself, enjoy this period of celebration. DATE NIGHT is a ritual.

You had a great week. Now's the time to either create a romantic meal at home, order pizza, make a favorite treat, or go to a party!

STOCK UP!
TEN-et Seven

7 Days of Dinners, Planned & Purchased

The seventh lifestyle essential of *Light Ten Up!* is important and very counter-cultural. The goal here is to plan dinner one week in advance, and purchase what you will need for the whole week. When you *stock up*, you will be rid of the daily choice at the heart of the most loathsome sentence in the English language: "*What's for dinner?*"

People do not plan to fail, but when we fail to plan the whole day's nutrition, we get to the end of our rope and eat poorly. Does this sound familiar? You go all day counting calories, and then suddenly realize you have gone over budget. The whole day is shot, so you eat whatever is in the pantry. Think about it. How many times have you been sad that you ate all your allotted calories, and now dinner is only *celery*? Let's to do something different here, and plan dinner ahead of time, having the supper supplies on hand, ahead of time.

Every day of the week has a vibe. Along the ideas of ritual, order and ceremony, I recommend leaning into the vibe, and creating a theme for each night of the week.

Monday is meatless, to reduce our carbon footprint. Taco Tuesday is just *correct.* I mean, who doesn't love the Lego Movie reference? Wednesday is wacky, so keep the meal basic. The TV show *Friends* was the best part of the week, Thursday nights from 1994 to 2004, so I honor the vibe by making the chop salad the cast ate for lunch daily for ten years. *Could Jennifer Anniston BE any sexier*? Friday is fish, because I'm *Catholic-ish.* Saturday is DATE NIGHT, ceremonial to my marriage. And Sunday is so soulful that a pot of soup simmering in the kitchen is so Mmm-Mmmm good.

<u>Checklist for TEN-et Seven: STOCK UP!</u>

On Saturday, make a shopping list and head to the store. Each weekend, you will shop for the entire week's groceries, so you have supper supplies. Since breakfast, lunch and snack plans are probably easiest to contrive, let's focus on the real issue for most folks: *What is for dinner*?? I build my meals around themes for each night. Each day of the week has its own vibe, so I lean into it. *This is the order of things in my house.* We enjoy every night of the week like it's a special occasion. Again, think: ***ritual, order, and ceremony***.

- <u>Meatless Monday</u> – Enjoy a Boca Burger or black bean patty and steamed zucchini.
- <u>Taco Tuesday</u> – Enjoy seasoned ground turkey or chicken meat, lettuce, tomato and salsa.
- <u>Wacky Wednesday</u> – Enjoy simple chicken and veg such as chicken sausage and broccoli.
- *Friends* <u>Thursday</u> – It's Chop Salad the *Friends* cast members ate every day for 10 years!
- <u>Fish Friday</u> – Enjoy gluten-free fish nuggets, or simply cod and steamed broccolini. Yum!
- <u>Saturday is DATE NIGHT</u> – Roast a chicken, order pizza, dine out, or attend a party!
- <u>Soulful-Soup-Night Sunday</u> – Choose a stew or soup that stirs the soul, like carrot ginger.

REST UP!
TEN-et Eight

8 Hours of Sleep

The eighth lifestyle essential of *Light Ten Up!* is the magic supplement for your entire brain and body. The missing secret ingredient for rebalancing hormones, increasing the space between synapses, healing every organ, cell and system is sleep. Human growth hormone is a key component for lipolysis, the process by which fat cells are emptied. Sleep provides you with Human growth hormone. Quite simply, sleep helps you burn fat.

Deep inside all of us is a little kid who's not about to be told it's time for bed. The internet has too many fun things going on, and thanks to *The Social Dilemma*, you now know why you can't look away. The trick here, my dear friend, is to get up early in the morning, keep it moving all day long, and to practice the routine called *Wash Up and Wind Down*, two hours before bedtime.

<u>Checklist for TEN-et Eight: REST UP!</u>

- After Dinner, clean up the kitchen and close it. Turn off the lights, clean and dry the sink.
- Go wash your face. Bathe if you like. Brush and floss your teeth. Use your Listerine.
- Put on the highest quality best-feeling pajamas you can possibly afford. Treat yourself!
- Shuffle around in your PJ's and feel your blood pressure drop immediately. Feel the transformation. Again, the virtues of ritual, order and ceremony are important here.
- Avoid eating or drinking while in pajamas. Tempted? Use teeth whitening strips.
- Log off the internet, period. People in your life are ready to respect your boundaries.
- As you snuggle pets and loved ones, enjoy light television or light reading. No drama.
- As you shuffle around in your pajama luxury, turn off superfluous lights as you go.
- Essential oils in a diffuser are great for sleep. So are melatonin and Sleepy time Tea.

Friends, it can be challenging to prioritize sleeping 8 hours a night. Folks with children, stressful times and issues like sleep apnea can all add to the drama. Please refer to the tenets of sleep hygiene. Your bed is for sleeping, and not eating or playing video games, surfing the internet, or talking on the phone. Steps like investing in great pajamas and essential oils like clary sage and lavender can help.

Our culture celebrates productivity and pushing through, rather than sleeping eight hours. Resist the impulse to skimp. The hunger hormone ghrelin, and the satiety hormone leptin each balance out with optimal sleep. Have you ever noticed being hungrier on a day where you'd slept poorly that night? Sleep equals weight loss and weight maintenance.

Get up early, and power through a busy day every night of the week. Sleep comes easier this way. Conversely, sleeping in guarantees that you will not be able to fall asleep, come bedtime. Every morning, I leap out of bed at 3:30 a.m. before my 4 am alarm even goes off. I get up happily, knowing I will be very, very sleepy come 7:30 p.m. Sleeping eight hours every night is 100% why I am losing weight, getting to goal.

LIGHT IT UP!
TEN-et Nine

9 Minutes of Tai Chi'll

The ninth lifestyle essential of *Light Ten Up!* is a daily practice of Tai Chi that I have recently created. I call this tradition of movement and calming groove *Tai Chi'll*. I have been teaching Tai Chi as a certified BTS/ Les Mills International *Body Flow* teacher since 2003. Since 2017, I have practiced Tai Chi daily during daily long walks outdoors. I love having my headphones on and grooving to the form I learned from my Tai Chi teacher. As an experienced group fitness instructor with an eye towards fun, I took what I like about Tai Chi the martial art, and fashioned my own flowy, ecstatic dance experience. I've named my class Tai Chi'll because this is what I'm after: a fun, sustainable practice to heal my joints, calm my nerves, and chill the hell out. I love it.

Friends, this practice is great for relaxation and vitality, as well as for healing joints. For 5,000 years, Tai Chi has helped people stay healthy and agile, addressing blood sugar imbalances, stress, and heart disease. At 9 am, every day, you have a chance to stop, drop and do Tai Chi'll. I hope you like this fun group fitness class, using music and movement to improve balance, focus and to reduce anxiety. 9 am is a ceremonious moment in your day.

Assuming you are working from home, or in an office, or are raising a family, chances are that you are accountable to someone, or some project for which the agreed-upon start time is 9 am. This is a good time to align your life's path with a mindfulness moment, like Tai Chi'll.

I know it might sound counter-intuitive to add another thing to the list, but the return on your investment of 9 minutes at 9 am will be extraordinary.

The time of day isn't super important, but again, we employ ritual, order and ceremony to great effect here. At 9 am, you are shifting from your personal life to your professional life, typically. The activities we do prior to 9 am are typically for ourselves, and the activities we do after 9 am are typically for others and for the wider world. This transition deserves fanfare and, well *ceremony*. Tai Chi'll classes with me on YouTube will be a practice of ease and peace. Even joy.

I am describing a moment every day for you to take a deep breath and really inTENtionally step into your working day, on purpose with purpose. So much of life is hurry and go, and wait, and hurry more. We do not stop and smell the coffee, but race like rats to the big Nowhere, fast. At 9 am, you can take 9 minutes to get it together on purpose to great effect.

Your goal is not to get good at Tai Chi'll. Your goal is to use the practice to flip a switch in your brain. You'll switch from the mindset of "*I have to*" to "*I get to.*" It's that simple.

Let's check it out.

<u>Checklist for TEN-et Nine: LIGHT IT UP!</u>

- Find the latest offering of mine on YouTube – Open Up! With Danielle Day
- To begin, ask yourself: Who loves me? To whom do I dedicate my best? And how?
- Think about how awesome it is to have loved ones who want you to take care of yourself.
- Take a deep breath. Notice how great that feels. The abundance of air is everywhere.
- Think: How do I convert the air in my lungs to the effort I expend?
- Move easily and happily through the *Tai Chi'll* practice with these ideas in mind. Enjoy!

Tai Chi'll with Danielle Day works best with music. What's your favorite 5-minute song? You will learn how to mix and match the moves over time for your own independent practice.

This will be a wonderful activity to share with your kids, friends and family.

Tai Chi'll by Danielle Day: Look for it in group fitness classes everywhere soon, alongside aerobics classes for active older adults, (or **Classic Rockers***, as I call us).*

STEP IT UP!
TEN-et Ten

Ten Thousand Steps Per Day

The tenth lifestyle essential of *Light Ten Up!* is a daily goal. Congratulations, by the way on making it to the tenth essential. This step is associated with weight loss as well as weight management. Research proves that people who walk 10,000 steps a day are more likely to maintain weight loss. The research pioneered at 20/20 Lifestyles at PRO Sports Club, under the direction of Dr Mark Dedomenico proves that 10,000 daily steps are keys to both losing weight, maintaining weight loss, and for improving the A-1C levels in Type 2 diabetics and folks with Metabolic Syndrome X, or what we call pre-diabetes.

So much about weight management has to do with your metabolism. The resting metabolic rate is affected by weight loss. It's simple math. You burn five calories per kilogram of body weight, for every five liters of oxygen you consume. Heavier bodies burn more calories just by breathing in and out. Add to this a little trick your body plays too. When a person loses a significant amount of weight, their daily natural activity *actually slows down.*

Our bodies are so hard-wired to gain and keep weight on for survival, it's been proven that people who've lost a lot of weight naturally slow down all daily movement naturally. Basically, our modern bodies need to keep moving on purpose every day to keep the fire of the metabolism burning. The resting metabolic rate for each person varies, but research done at 20/20 demonstrates that all bodies will burn fewer calories after weight loss, in addition to a natural propensity to slow down physical movement.

When we have weight to lose, we burn a lot of calories naturally. When we have less weight, or no excess weight to lose, we do not burn as many. It's tough. The fitter you become, the more efficient your body becomes. It can be frustrating. Happily, you have technology now to track your steps, and to track how many calories you are burning through your movement.

My Apple Watch is my very best friend. I can set all kinds of timers to keep myself on track. I get to earn little rewards all day by meeting my Move, Stand and Exercise goals. You guys! This is important. You can have the most kick-ass workouts possible, but if you are sedentary the whole rest of the day, your health is seriously compromised. The slow burn all day of a moving body is what you are aiming for. 10,000 steps are the minimum!

<u>Checklist for TEN-et Ten: STEP IT UP!</u>

- Get a walk outside, rain or shine every single day. Plan to do this after Yoga or Weights.
- Walk for 40 minutes before you take your morning shower.
- Use very comfortable shoes. I love Sketchers with the memory foam in them.
- Bring headphones and your smartphone. Listen to podcasts!
- My podcast is ***Light Not Might***. New episodes drop on Mondays.
- Aim for a goal to burn half as many calories as you'll eat all day, through movement, including walking, yoga, and lifting weights.

Example: my resting metabolic rate is 1,300. My Naturopathic Doctor has calculated this. My goal is to eat 1,200 calories daily. Already, this helps me be deficient by 100 calories daily. My Move Goal is 600 calories. This helps me to be deficient by 700 calories daily. This caloric deficit multiplied by five to seven days a week leaves me deficient in caloric intake by 3,500 calories minimum. There are 3,500 calories in one pound of excess body fat, or adipose tissue. I lose about one pound a week.

I can maintain this loss with 10,000 steps per day.

Exercise definitely helps me achieve my Move Goal of 600 calories. My 10,000 Steps goal will combat any decrease in my natural activity all day. I definitely notice myself sitting more when I'm losing weight. My friends and family often comment on my affect. I even speak slower and sit more still and quietly when I am losing weight. My body obviously likes to add pounds and not let them go. I easily go up and down 60 pounds or more when I am not practicing the Ten Essential Steps to Glow By. Thank you for listening. I'm excited to share what I practice.

STARTING UP!
Putting Light Ten Up! into practice.

Congratulations again, on joining me on the path to your very best. Now that you've read the *Ten Lifestyle Essentials to Glow By*, we can explore the big ideas a little more in depth, as to their application. My goal is to help you create a lifestyle that involves the ritual, order and ceremony we've explored in the *Ten Lifestyle Essentials to Glow By*. In this section, you will find a list of things to have on hand, as well as shopping lists, recipes and a few thoughts on how to structure your day for optimal results.

Feeling overwhelmed? Remember, you are on a path a little like hiking the Appalachian Trail. At first, you get a guide, a map, and your gear together. Then it's just a matter of putting one foot in front of the other until you get there. Remember that simply taking action counts. You are in it for the long haul, so please feel good that you are not on a diet. Rather, you are restructuring your schedule and tweaking your priorities to align with your vision. Very soon the results you seek will appear.

SHOW UP!
Time Management

The most important service a lifestyle coach can offer is coaching your time management. I am personally obsessed with time. Years ago, when I was a new runner, training for my first marathon, I read The Women's Book of Running. The author made a point that served me very well as a working mom with a small child. She said that time was a finite resource, and that the most important strategy in life was to make the clock your friend. As an athlete, she was battling the clock to improve her speed. But as a woman, she said she was using time as the ultimate tool for getting what she wanted out of life.

Although I have forgotten the exact title of the book, and the dear author's name, I will never forget her saying, "Running is the canvas upon which I paint my very best life." I think about these words every time I run. I will never forget challenging myself to the 5k route around our neighborhood, leaving exactly 30 minutes before my daughter's school bus would bring her home from elementary school. My goal was a ten-minute mile, so the 3.2 miles around the hood and back was important. The specter of my first-grader locked out of our house because her mom was indulging in a workout was enough to make me run fast! I treasure the memories of her waving at me from the school bus window as I raced to beat her school bus home.

The word Time needs a capital T because it is the most valuable resource you have. Think is like wealth. Time is the most valuable and irreplaceable resource of your life. Think about it. Steve Jobs and Paul Allen, for all their combined billions could not purchase what you are afforded every day you wake up. My mother passed away eight years ago, and as I get closer and closer each year to the age she was when she was diagnosed with Stage 4 breast cancer, I am keenly aware that life is a precious gift. My beloved dog passed away in my arms after thirteen years of joy and love. When it's over, it's really over. Time is precious and irreplaceable.

When you wake up in the morning, avoid picking up your phone. Stop. Breathe. Feel the sheets on your skin. Listen to the breathing of the partner next to you, pets beside you, or just the sense of safety and peace around you. Stop and say thank you. I am not aware of your spiritual inclinations, but I feel like we can all get our heads around the memo that life is not a problem to push through. Life is not a pile of Have-To. Life is a pile of Get-To. This is the essence of self-care. If you do not feel more blessed than you do stressed, then please take action. There is a choice you can make to feel grateful. That's the coach in me talking, and it's the most important thing I think I can say. Thank you for listening.

Daily we begin with lifestyle essential Number One: ***First Thing's First***. The first priority of every day is your twenty-minute planning session. As you practice entering your food strategy for the day, it will get faster and easier. The app I use is Nutritionix because it's very trainable. Since I practice lifestyle essential Number Seven (Seven Days of Dinners), the app knows what my food choices are going to be, simply because of the day of the week. I can whip through this step so fast now. The next step, as you know, is to schedule the appointments with yourself for your workouts. 60 minutes for Yoga, or Weights, and 40 minutes for a walk outdoors. Yes, I said AND. You have two workouts Monday through Friday. The weekends are a little more flexible for grocery shopping, DATE NIGHT and Family Time.

There are 24 hours in every day. Let's say, ten of these hours are devoted to Work. Whether you are making a home, working a job, looking for work (which is then a job you are doing like a job), let's assume work takes 10 hours of your daily 24.

I worked three jobs for a year, when I weighed 123 pounds. I was a single mom with a teenager at that point, and worked at PRO Club from 5 am to 3 pm, then stopped off and met a client to personally train her, on my way to my Starbucks' Corporate fitness job called **Kinetix** *from 4 to 9 pm. I taught hot yoga classes on the weekends and I even traveled 3 hours from Seattle to Portland on alternate weekends to date the man is who now my husband. I know busy. You too can manage time well. After all, look at all you have accomplished in your life!*

Lifestyle essential number eight of course, takes eight hours for sleeping. This is non-negotiable. As you know, the human body will not burn fat, repair itself, organize brain activity and support your immune system unless you rest. So that is eight hours.

Given that eighteen hours are spoken for, that leaves six for living. In the lifestyle we are working on here, **two hours** are for exercise and planning Monday through Friday. (Saturday is an hour for grocery shopping and the twenty minutes in the morning for planning. Sunday is twenty minutes in the morning for planning, and hopefully you schedule an hour for an active Family Time.) *I'm calling this "Two for you, 'Boo".* There are six hours in the day where you are not working or sleeping. *Of this six, claim two for you.* **TWO.**

You are scheduling two hours for yourself each day. You can use the calendar on your phone, but I am old-school. I love handwriting in journals because I save them. In the future, if I fall out of practice with the ten essentials, I can then "time-travel" back to a period when I was living at my best. I get support from a better version of myself.

Recall Lifestyle Essential Number One: *First Thing's First.* You have a finite number of calories you get to eat each day. It's a budget. Similarly, you have a finite amount of time in which to get funky. Carving out two hours for your lifestyle each day **is the lifestyle**. *Two for You, 'Boo.* Still feeling like that is not achievable? Let's talk.

My degree is in Sociology, with an emphasis in Social Work. In my career, I have counseled people in every setting from weight loss, to credit counseling, to surviving domestic violence. One thing is constant in every setting: *start where the client is.* Your personal ability to manage time is what got you this far in life, so take heart. You can do anything you feel is important to you. But what if you can't *because of other people*?

Boundaries are important in life. You have people you care for, and take care of, and would *do anything for.* What happens when those same people are not choosing to support your lifestyle goals? If it's your kids, then find ways to incorporate lifestyle into your life as a family. My favorite Ironman Triathlon client would bring her seven-year-old son and his bike along, on our long runs. We got in our mileage, and she parented the heck out of this amazing young person.

Friends, I cannot think of anything more educational than crunching numbers as a family, with regards to calories and meal planning. As a child, shopping with my own single mother and three siblings was a weekly ritual. We were all responsible for making the shopping list, then working to adhere to mom's budget. We all played a part in the shopping. On payday, there was pizza. (DATE NIGHT!)

Time is your right. Time belongs to you. Who is *taking,* more than *giving*? Are they threatened by your taking charge of your lifestyle? Trust me. In my job at Jenny Craig Weight Loss Centers, we saw this kind of thing all the time. Sadly, in my career as a Domestic Violence Woman's Advocate, it was also a common theme. Heck, even in yoga teacher training I saw this kind of dynamic play out. When you step up your game, folks in your life can become triggered.

My encouragement to you, in response to people who are threatened by your lifestyle makeover, is to simply smile and say, "*I am so grateful that I can count on you to support my goals.*"

As your coach, it is my honor to hold space for you. I can help you to role-play any sticky scenarios. There are no judgements. Only tips, tricks and strategies. Losing weight shifts the power dynamic in any relationship. It rocks the boat! As your coach, I am here to help you navigate any choppy waters ahead.

LIVE IT UP!
Date Night!

When I deprive myself of the things I want, I tend not to stick to my goals. I encourage you, dear reader, to think of the foods and beverages that you really want to incorporate into a balanced lifestyle. Think of the notion of gateway foods. Each of us has a *kryptonite* kind of food. Is there something against which you are typically powerless? For me, it is sourdough bread. I cannot stop eating sourdough bread! What is a category of foods that you just know you need to say *goodbye for now* to?

What are the foods you love AND that we can incorporate into your plan?

One great moment in the week when you can enjoy your favorite treats is Saturday night. We call this DATE NIGHT because we are leveraging ritual, order and ceremony to great effect.

Let's look at the slate of options for Saturday Night:

Date Night.

- Roasted chicken at home. At 425 degrees, it takes less than two hours to roast a chicken for you to serve as a romantic meal at the table, with leftovers from Sunday to Wednesday!

- DATE NIGHT out at a restaurant, once a month for a special birthday or fun night out.

- Pizza Night! This is America. You simply must have pizza at least monthly. Right?!

- Product Night. We all have something like Annie's Organic Mac and Cheese in the cupboard. Monthly, why not enjoy this incredibly satisfying meal? Add your favorite toppings. YUM

EAT UP!
My eating strategy

Breakfast is coffee and eggs, on Sundays with bacon.

Lunch is always a salad with the *Friends* recipe in mind, or dinner leftovers.

Dinners are planned ahead of time, honoring a theme for each day of the week.

Variety is key. I enjoy Soup on Sundays, so that is the wild card for ingredients.

I shop on Saturday, so I look for a delightful recipe to simmer on the stove or cook in the crock pot. It is all about seasonal ingredients and variety.

Gazpacho in summer, Stew in winter, or Carrot Ginger! *So Romantic*.

WHIP IT UP!
Recipes

Friends' Chop Salad
Jennifer Aniston's Favorite

1 cup cooked bulghur

2 peeled and seeded diced cucumbers

1 15 ounce can of garbanzo beans, rinsed and drained

¼ cup minced red onion

2 Tablespoons chopped fresh parsley

1 Tablespoon chopped fresh mint

½ cup crumbled fresh feta cheese

½ cup shelled pistachios

Toss it up and serve with lemon slices, salt and pepper to taste!

Store in airtight container in the fridge. It lasts, since there is no dressing!

Coach Danielle's Perfect Crustless Cheesecake!

4 8-ounce bricks of cream cheese, softened to room temperature

2 eggs, also at room temperature

1 cup SWERVE Confectioners style sugar substitute

¼ cup sour cream

1 Tbsp. sugarfree vanilla flavor (such as Torani syrup)

1 tsp. pure vanilla extract

1 tsp. pure lemon extract

Combine everything until it's very smooth. Pour into prepared springform pan.

Place into 350-degree oven and bake 30-35 minutes. It will be jiggly when you take it out. Place on the counter to cool thoroughly, then cover and place in the refrigerator overnight. Each slice has 3 net carbs, 326 calories, 26 grams of fat, and 9 grams of protein.

PRO Tip: I budget one slice every day for myself. If I end up eating a little more of my other food choices that day, and it looks like I won't meet my calorie target of 1,200, then I will enjoy a half slice or less of sugar free cheesecake that day. Following Lifestyle Essential Number One, I include one slice of this treat in my daily plan. That way, I get cheesecake. Plus, I can tweak how much of one slice I actually get, depending on my adherence to my overall daily plan. Nibble at something off plan? I take a smaller portion of cheesecake later that day. Mess up altogether? No cheesecake.

I bake one cheesecake every weekend! It's part of my romantic Saturday night cooking.

Danielle's Taco Tuesday Salad

1 pound ground chicken or turkey meat

1 tsp cayenne pepper

1 tsp cumin

Romaine lettuce leaves

Two roma tomatoes

1 Tbsp Salsa

1 Tbsp sour cream

2 T grated sharp cheddar cheese. Chipotle cheese, if we have it on hand!

1 Tbsp olive oil.

One packet of Hidden Valley Spicy Ranch salad dressing/ seasoning mix

Heat the olive oil in your Dutch oven or pan until shimmery. Add the pound of ground chicken meat. Season with light salt and pepper. Go easy on salt. Add the cayenne, cumin and seasoning packet. Cook until meat temperature reaches 165. Take off the heat, place in a cool bowl and let it cool. Chop your romaine, tomatoes, and shred your cheese. Make your dressing: mix the salsa and the sour cream in a little dish. Toss the dressing with the veggies, add 3 ounces of the chicken mixture, top with shredded cheese. As with the Chop Salad recipe, I'll let you plug your exact portions into Nutritionix for the calorie total. Enjoy! Such a yummy Tuesday dinner

GATHER UP!
Grocery Shopping

Each week, I visit the supermarket closest to my house. My practice is to shop only one time per week. This presents a challenge, but pretty much guarantees that I stay on top of things.

For me, I get into mischief when I visit the store multiple times in a week. When I am "up to no good", as I like to say, I will invent a reason to run to the store, like, **we are low on cat food**, *and then I'll buy something off-plan, like ice cream or a can of wine. So classy, I know.*

When I am on plan, following *the ten lifestyle essentials*, I make a shopping list all throughout the week, organized around my themes for dinner. There are staples that we always need, and when I grab it all in a one-hour round trip to the store, I only keep what I need (and very little of what I crave) in my home.

Shopping once a week is my ritual. There is order and ceremony to the whole process, including a gratitude prayer when I pay at the counter. Thank You, Universe for all the money we have so we can eat well. Thank you for food.

Speaking of money, you also save money when you only shop once a week. There is an industry calculation I heard once that for every minute you spend in the store, you grab $5 worth of things. I take about 40 minutes, so that sounds about right. Plus, by dining out once a month, and only doing takeout food once a month, our budget is happy too.

My Sample Shopping List:

- Romaine lettuce, 2 cucumbers, 2 zucchini, 1 broccolini, red onion, celery
- Mint, parsley, basil, garlic, ginger root, 2 tomatoes, 1 avocado, limes
- Eggs, bacon, turkey bacon, string cheese, cream cheese, sour cream
- One whole organic chicken, Aidel's chicken sausages, cod, ground chicken
- Feta cheese, kalmata olives, Newman's Own Oil and Vinegar dressing
- Hint waters- 7 one for each day to put in my 4 liters of water
- Alcohol of choice
- Coffee, Tea and Torani sugar free syrup
- SWERVE. The best sugar substitute in the world.
- Boca Burgers, frozen veggies, Newman's Own Pizza as needed
- Sparkling waters: Pellegrino, Perrier, La Croix, Topo Chico, Gerolsteiner
- Cat Food and whatever toiletries and paper supplies we need.

GEAR UP!
Things you will need

Here are things that are a must-have, in addition to a smartphone.

- Food Scale. You have to measure your food to track your nutrition.
- People Scale. You have to measure your body so you can track progress.
- Bath Gloves. These are exfoliating and available at the drugstore.
- Dry Brush. This can be a little harder to find, so try Whole Foods. Fancy!
- Highest Quality Pajamas you can possibly afford. Seriously. A MUST.
- Yoga Mat. You can buy an awesome Gaiam mat at the drugstore too.
- Dumbells in large, medium & small, such as 12-20 lbs, 8-10 lbs and 3-5 lbs.
- A small measuring cup that gets down to ounces. Very handy.
- Springform pan if you plan to make cheesecake.

Apps for your smartphone

- Rep Count
- Nutritionix
- YouTube
- Podcast app, such as Apple Podcasts or Spotify
- Pedometer

LEVEL UP!
Personal Coaching

Thank you for taking the time to read *Light Ten Up, Ten Lifestyle Essential to Glow By*.

I'd love to coach you. All my life I have struggled to really find the routine that was going to do the trick. I have always wanted to find the balanced lifestyle that would afford me the chance to look my best while enjoying my favorite things. I am sure this program is it.

As you can see, this program is all about structure and routine, or what I lovingly call *ritual, order and ceremony*. It is about putting self-monitoring, tracking, measuring and moving up front. If you are in the place where you would like the support, and the genuine human connection, then I would love to coach you.

My email address is **Danielle@openupyogatt.com** Reach out anytime, please. Thanks!

I am especially looking forward to training my Yoga Teacher Training alumni to become Lifestyle Coaches too. Please join the movement at *Light Ten Up*! We have a Facebook page, and a private group for folks on the path. My podcast "***Light Not Might***" is also available for the inspiration!

Friends, to each their own journey. I affirm your worth and your dignity just as you are.

Thank you for listening.

You're awesome! D.D.

READ UP!
Works of Inspiration and Guidance

Abhedananda, S. (1967). *The Yoga Psychology.* Calcutta: Ramakrishna Vedanta Math.

Akers, B. D. (2002). *Hatha Yoga Pradipika, The Original Sanskrit Svatmarama.* Woodstock, New York: YogaVidya.com.

Anodea, J. (1996). *Eastern Body, Western Mind: Psychology and the Chakra System as a Path to the Self.* Celestial Arts.

Bachman, N. (2004). *Language of Yoga.* Boulder, CO: Sounds True, Inc.

Baptiste, B. (2002). *Journey into Power.* New York, NY: Simon and Schuster, NY.

Barnett, M. (2004). *Hot Yoga.* Hauppauge NY: Barrons Educational Series, Inc.

Birch, B. B. (1995). *Power Yoga.* New York, NY: Fireside Books.

BKS Iyengar and Silva, M. a. (1990). *Yoga the Iyengar Way.* U.S.: Alfred A Knopf, Inc.

Broad, W. J. (2012). *The Science of Yoga: The Risks and Rewards.* New York: Simon & Schuster.

Brooks, R. (Director). (1958). *Cat on a Hot Tin Roof* [Motion Picture].

Byrne, R. (2012). *The Magic.* New York, NY: Atria Books.

Carrera, R. J. (2006). *Inside the Yoga Sutras.* Buckingham, VA: Integral Yoga Publications.

Chatlani, M. (2003). *Yoga Flows.* London, UK: Carroll and Brown Publishers.

Chinmayananda, S. (1959). *The Sreemad-Bhagawad-Geeta.* Madras, India: The Chinamaya Publication Trust.

Choudhury, B. (1978). *Bikrams Beginning Yoga Class.* New York, NY: GP Penguin/Putnams Sons.

Clark, B. (2012). *The Complete Guide to Yin Yoga.* Ashland, OR: White Cloud Press.

Cope, S. (1999). *Yoga and the Quest for the True Self.* New York, NY: Bantam Books.

Costill, J. H. (1994). *Phyiology of Sport and Exercise.* Champagne, Illinois: Human Kinetics.

DeBell, R. (2018). *Movement Fix.* Retrieved from themovementfix.com: http://www.themovementfix.com

Desikachar, T. (1995). *The Heart of Yoga.* Rochester, VT: Inner Traditions, International.

Docter, P. (Director). (2015). *Inside Out!* [Motion Picture].

Dr Sylvia Tara, P. (2016). *The Secret Life of Fat.* New York, New York: Penguin Random House Books.

Eliade, M. (1975). *Patanjali and Yoga.* New York, NY: Schocken Books.

Farhi, D. (2000). *Yoga Mind, Body and Spirit.* New York, New York: Holt Paperbacks.

Farhi, D. (2000). *Yoga Mind, Body and Spirit.* New York, New York: Holt Paperbacks.

Faulds, R. (2006). *Kripalu Yoga.* New York, NY: Bantam Dell.

Gannon, D. L. (2011). *Jivamukti Yoga.* Ballantine Books.

Georg Feuerstein, P. (1998). *The Yoga Tradition.* Prescott ,Arizona: Hohm Press.

Gibran, K. (1973). *The Prophet.* New York, NY: Alfred A Knopf.

Goss, C. S. (1959). *Yoga for Today.* New York, NY: Holt Reinhart and Winston.

Grilley, P. (2012). *Yin Yoga, Principles and Practice.* Ashland, OR: White Cloud Press.

Gundry, D. S. (2018). *The Plant Paradox Cookbook: 100 Recipes to Help You Lose Weight, Heal Your Gut and Live Lectin-Free.* New York, : Harper Collins.

Hewitt, J. (1977). *The Complete Yoga.* New York, NY: Schocken Books.

Hittleman, R. (1969). *28 Day Exercise Plan.* New York, NY: Bantam Dell.

Houston, Y., & M.A. (n.d.). *The Yoga Sutra Workbook, The Certainty of Freedom.* American Sanskrit Institute.

Iyengar, B. (1966). *Light on Yoga.* New York, NY: Schocken Books.

Iyengar, B. (2003). *Light on Life.* Rodale, Inc.

Iyengar, B. (2005). *Light on Life.* United States of America: Rodale.

Jagannathan, V. (2015). *Yoga in Visishtadvaita.* Charleston, South Carolina: Self Published.

Johnson, C. (2012). *The Yoga Sutras of Patanjali.* Digireads.com Books.

Juan Ramon Jimenez, t. b. (1973). *I Am Not I.* Beacon Press.

Judith Lasater, P. P. (2004). *Yoga for Pregnancy.* Berkeley, California: Rodmell Press, Yoga Shorts.

Kaminoff, L. (2007). *Yoga Anatomy.* Champagne IL: Human Kinetics.

Kissiah, G. (n.d.). *The Yoga Sutras of Patanjali.* Lila Labs Publishing, LLC.

Kittel C. Kroemer, H. (1980). *Thermal Physics.* San Francisco.

Lee, C. (2004). *Yoga Body, Buddha Mind.* New York, NY: The Berkley Publishing Group.

Little, T. (2003). *Sthira Sukham Asanam.* Santa Fe, New Mexico: Yogasource.

Long, R. M. (2005). *The Key Muscles of Yoga*. Bandha Yoga Publications, LLC.

Long, R. M. (2008). *The Key Poses of Yoga*. Bandha Yoga Publications, LLC.

Luby, S. (1974). *Yoga is for You*. Englewood Cliffs, NJ: Prentice Hall, Inc.

MacDonald, G. (1892). *British Quaker Periodical*.

Marieb, E. N. (2002). *Anatomy & Physiology*. San Fransisco : Benjamin Cummings.

McTaggart, L. (2008). *The Field*. New York, NY: Harper.

Meza, M. (2007). *Art of Sequencing- a Yoga Instructional*. Seattle, Washington: Melina Meza Press.

Mitchell, S. (2000). *The Bhagavad Gita*. New York NY: Three Rivers Press.

Mithoefer, B. (2006). *The Yin Yoga Kit*. Rochester, VT: Healing Arts Press.

Muzumdar, S. (1949). *Yogic Exercises*. Calcutta: Orient Longmans Private Ltd.

Myss, C. P. (1997). *Anatomy of the Spirit*. Harmony.

Nietzsche, F. (1882). *The Parable of the Madman*.

Norberg, U. (2014). *Yin Yoga*. New York, New York: Skyhorse Publishing, Inc.

Pandit Rajmanitigunait, P. (2014). *The Secret of the Yoga Sutras Samadhi Pada*. Honesdale, PA: Himalayan Institute.

Piaget, J. (1977). Piaget's Theory of Cognitive Development. *The role of action in the development of thinking.*, 17-42.

Picozzi, M. (1998). *Pocket Guide to Hatha Yoga*. Berkeley, California: The Crossing Press.

Pollan, M. (2007). *The Omnivore's Dilemma a Natural* . United States of America: Penguin Books.

Prabhavananda, S. (1948). *The Upanishads Breath of the Eternal*. New York, New York: Penguin Books.

Ravindran, R. (n.d.). Yoga 108. *i-phone ap.* support@yoga108app.com.

Reis, J. (2012). *Divine Sleep*.

Sara Santarossa, J. L. (2017). #Orthorexia on Instagram: A Descriptive Study Exploring the Online Conversation and Community Using Netlytic Software. *Eating and Weight Disorders*.

Singhal, J. (2009). *Yoga Perceived and Practised*. Jawahar Nagar, NewDelhi: Raman Chaudhary.

Singhal, J. (2009). *Yoga Perceived and Practised*. Jawar Nagar, New Dehli: Raman Chaudhary.

Sivananda, S. S. (1978). *The Science of PrAnayama*. Himalayas India: The Divine Life Society.

Stephens, M. (2012). *Yoga Sequencing*. Berkeley, California: North Atlantic Books.

Stone, M. (2008). *The Inner Tradition of Yoga*. Boston, Mass.: Shambhala Publications.

Taimni, I. (1961). *The Science of Yoga*. Wheaton, IL: The Theosophical Publishing House.

Taylor, D. J. (2008). *My Stroke of Insight*. New York: Viking Penguin.

Thoreau, H. D. (August 9, 1854). *Walden; or, Life in the Woods*. Boston, Massachusetts : Ticknor and Fields.

Tzu, L. (6th-century BC). *Tao Te Ching*. China (Zhou).

Vig, B. (Director). (2014). *Sonic Highways* [Motion Picture].

Vishnudevananda, S. (1960). *The Complete Illustrated Book of Yoga*. New York, NY: Bell Publishing Company, Inc.

PICK IT UP!
Links

Light Not Might Podcast - https://anchor.fm/lightnotmight

Open Up Yoga Teacher Training - https://www.openupyogatt.com/

Teaching Yoga: The Side Hustle to Save the World -
    https://amzn.to/2LMhaCM

YouTube - https://www.youtube.com/c/OpenUpwithDanielleDay/

Hatha Yoga Class - Leaving Bikram - https://youtu.be/FNtpJHxi0TE

8 Minute Abs - https://youtu.be/g9jBjFTBF3A

Dry Brush Technique - https://youtu.be/CvxNDjVveWE

About the Author

Danielle Day is an expert yoga teacher trainer living on the North Shore of Lake Washington, in Seattle. She lives with her beloved husband and pets, celebrating the successful life of her young adult daughter. Living, loving, and enjoying the empty-nesting years, Danielle is embracing a post-Covid career pivot. Incorporating ten years in Social Work, ten years in Personal Training, and ten years in Yoga Teacher Training, Danielle is a certified lifestyle coach with a unique skillset.

Committed to starting where her client is, Danielle is well-equipped to serve every kind of person, from weight loss clients to triathletes and marathoners. *Light Ten Up*! is Danielle's impassioned offering to the wider world, as a testament to the healing power of fitness, nutrition, and genuine human connection.

Follow Danielle on her podcast **Light Not Might**, her YouTube Channel **Open Up! with Danielle Day**, and her website, **OpenUpYogaTT.com**. There, you'll find links to her other books, such as **"Teaching Yoga. The Side-Hustle to Save the World"** available on Amazon.

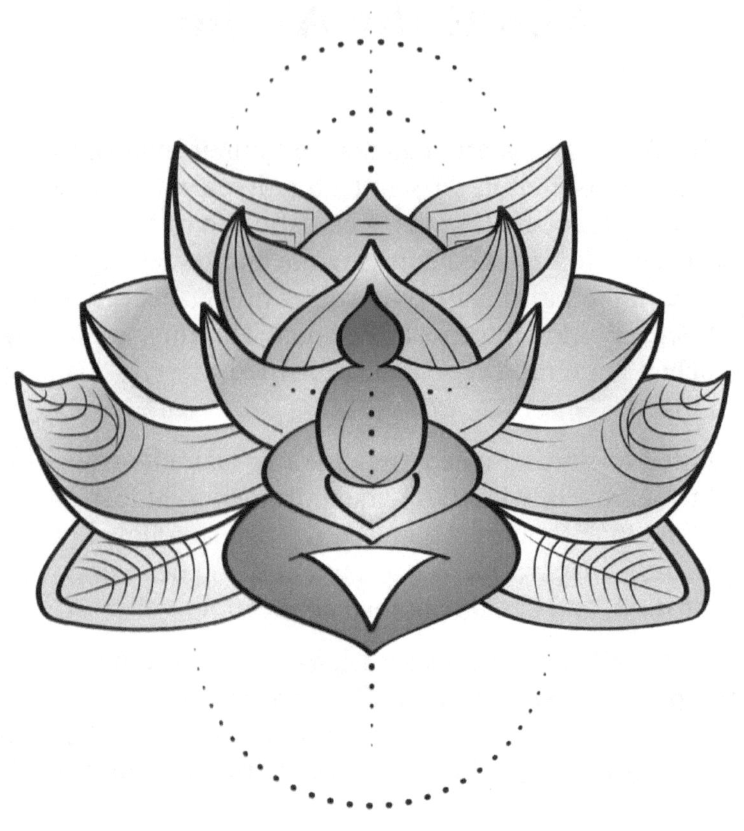